C000212063

TOP TIPS

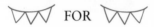 FOR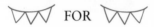

NEW PARENTS

VERITY DAVIDSON

summersdale

TOP TIPS FOR NEW PARENTS

An Hachette UK Company
www.hachette.co.uk

Summersdale Publishers Ltd
Part of Octopus Publishing Group Limited
Carmelite House
50 Victoria Embankment
LONDON
EC4Y 0DZ
UK

www.summersdale.com

Printed and bound in China

ISBN: 978-1-78685-973-0

Substantial discounts on bulk quantities of Summersdale books are available to corporations, professional associations and other organizations. For details contact general enquiries: telephone: +44 (0) 1243 771107 or email: enquiries@summersdale.com.

Disclaimer
The information given in this book should not be treated as a substitute for qualified medical advice. Neither the author nor the publisher can be held responsible for any loss or claim arising out of the use, or misuse, of the suggestions made or the failure to take medical advice.

With thanks to The Lullaby Trust.

CONTENTS

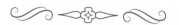

INTRODUCTION

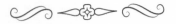

Congratulations, you're having a baby! There are exciting times ahead and this book will provide you with tips and insights to help you through those first few months. For first-time parents, the impending arrival of a baby, while a joyous event to look forward to, can be a little overwhelming. You might feel there is so much information to take in that you can't possibly retain it all – but don't panic! You will become a sponge

to all things baby and find you
have soaked up more information
than you realized, pulling it out
of the bag when you need it the
most. It's how we humans work.
So read on for tips on how
to prepare for your baby's
arrival, from practical to-do
and equipment lists, to how to
up your organization and when
to ask for help – plus advice
on how to care for, soothe and
feed your baby, how to do it all
on a budget, and tips on how
best to look after yourself too.
This is a new chapter of your life
and a great adventure awaits.

PREPARING FOR THE NEW ARRIVAL

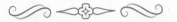

It pays to be organized before
your baby arrives. Make sure
you have all the kit ready and
the jobs done so you can put
your feet up for a well-earned
rest – it might be a while before
you get some of that again!

Every baby born into
the world is a finer
one than the last.

Charles Dickens

GETTING YOUR HOME READY

While you won't yet have to worry about stair gates, cupboard safety catches and applying padding to every corner in your home – it will be a good while before your baby is able to move about – there is still a certain amount of prep needed. Aside from the equipment you will require (see pp.12–16), think about where your baby will sleep. It is advised that they sleep in their parents' room for the first six months, so make sure you have the space to accommodate them – think practically and perhaps rethink the layout of your bedroom. Perhaps you want to get the nursery ready ahead of the baby's arrival so it's one less thing to worry about when the time comes for them to upgrade to their own room. Get any painting done ahead of time to avoid nasty fumes once the baby is with you (make sure any paints you use are safe for pregnant mums-to-be too); and look into the various pieces of furniture you might want, from a cot, which is essential unless you want to co-sleep (see page 120 for The Lullaby Trust's guidelines on safe co-sleeping), to the nice-to-have but less vital items such as a changing table, nursing chair, blackout blinds and perhaps somewhere to store the baby's things.

GATHERING YOUR EQUIPMENT TOGETHER

The list of kit you may think you need to buy can look a bit startling at first, but it really boils down to some basic essentials and then some optional and potentially useful extras. You're most likely already being spammed with various baby products and brands via social media – try not to pay them too much attention! Most of what these companies claim to be "must-haves" for newborns will be redundant after the first few weeks or months and most new parents get by perfectly well without them. You might be keen to buy brand new products for your brand new baby but, depending on your choices, some of these items can carry a hefty price tag. There are bargains to be had if you take the second-hand route via online auction and social media sites. See page 12 for the equipment essentials and the items it would be nice to have but you could easily do without.

THE EQUIPMENT ESSENTIALS

The must-haves:

◆ Baby car seat (you won't be able to safely transport the baby home from the hospital without one)

◆ Moses basket and/or crib for the first six months, plus bedding and/or a sleeping bag

◆ Pram, pushchair or "travel system" suitable for newborn upwards

◆ Cot, plus mattress and bedding (they will need this from six months so you can always buy it later)

- Newborn nappies and wipes
- Changing mat
- Breast pads
- Plenty of bibs
- Plenty of muslin squares
- Six long-sleeved baby suits
- Six short-sleeved baby suits
- Two cardigans
- Hat, mittens and booties
- Pramsuit or snowsuit (weather dependent)
- Nail scissors or clippers
- Digital thermometer

Children make you
want to start life over.

Muhammad Ali

The nice-to-haves:

- **Feeding equipment** – depending on the choice you've made about feeding your baby, you might need bottles, extra teats, sterilizing equipment, formula, a breast pump and so on; and, if you're breastfeeding, then a lanolin nipple cream is a *must*, and you may find nipple shields are a real help too.

- **Baby bath** – although you may find you can easily make do with your standard bath or a washing-up bowl.

- **Nappy bin** – these can be great for disposing of nappies, but you certainly pay a premium, with the bag refills costing a pretty penny!

◆ **Baby monitor** – the market is saturated: you can choose from the standard sound-only models to those that feature video, temperature and motion sensors.

◆ **Changing bag** – to keep your essentials organized when out and about, although a rucksack will do.

◆ **Sling/baby carrier** – if you want to try "babywearing" and leave the pram at home.

◆ **Bouncy chair** – so you can safely put your baby down and get on with other things.

◆ **Bath thermometer** – although many find the "elbow test" works just as well.

You can learn many
things from children.
How much patience
you have, for instance.

FRANKLIN P. JONES

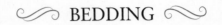

BEDDING

As well as having your Moses basket and/or crib ready, you'll need plenty of bedding essentials. The Lullaby Trust advises you to avoid bulky blankets and pillows as these might inadvertently end up tangled in your baby's limbs or covering their face. Rather, choose a firmly tucked-in sheet and blanket, below shoulder height, or a well-fitting sleeping bag. Make sure the neck hole of the sleeping bag is the right size so it will not slip over baby's head – if it does you will need a smaller size for now. If your Moses basket or crib is second-hand, you will need to buy a new mattress – this also applies if you have a second child, as these should always be fresh for each baby. According to The Lullaby Trust, the mattress should either have a waterproof cover or you should use sheets or a mattress protector with a water-resistant lining, to prevent any bodily fluids from seeping into the mattress itself and to help stop bacteria from accumulating. Choose from foam or organic wool/natural fibre and make sure it adheres to safety standards. The mattress shouldn't be too soft – it needs to offer your baby good support and a flat surface on which to sleep. As well as two sleeping bags or bedding sets (you may find that one is permanently in the wash!), you will also need at least two sheets to fit the mattress snugly.

SIGN UP FOR
∽ ANTENATAL ∾
CLASSES

There are lots of classes to choose from when it comes to learning how to care for your baby, helping you to be prepared for what to expect at the hospital when you arrive and for swotting up on how to handle those early days after your baby has been born. These tend to be available during the third trimester of pregnancy. Ask your midwife, health visitor or doctor about free antenatal classes in your local area or look into one of the many paid courses available. A little research will uncover a wealth of options, including those that incorporate hypnobirthing ideals and are more open-minded about alternative childbirth options such as home birth and birthing centres. A big plus when it comes to signing up to a course is that it's likely you will see the same faces each week, you will all be at roughly the same stage in your pregnancy and, once the babies arrive, you will have some comrades with whom to exchange nappy-related horror stories and sympathetic words about sleepless nights. And, once your baby is old enough, they will have other children their age to interact and play with.

PLANNING AHEAD

Now is the time to get organized and take advantage of the nesting instinct that will no doubt kick in. A couple of months before the baby is due, have a big clear-out and either sell or donate to charity the things you don't want or need any more. Get those niggling DIY jobs done (or arrange for professionals to sort these out for you) while you still can and before you're less mobile. A month before the due date give the house a deep clean and try to stay on top of tidying in the weeks that follow. Cleaning and tidying are likely to take a back seat once you have a new baby on your hands. A few weeks before your due date, batch cook lots of different meals that can be frozen, and divide them into portions before freezing so that simply defrosting and reheating will be a breeze. Think soup, lasagne, casserole, curry – or whatever you think will bring comfort in the early days. You'll thank yourself for your organization when you're feeling sleep-deprived and can only just about muster the energy to set the timer on the microwave. Another good tip is to get lots of early nights and nap whenever you possibly can – while you still can.

PACKING YOUR HOSPITAL BAG

You should pack your hospital bag 36 weeks into your pregnancy and keep it in an easily accessible place. You might need to leave your home in a hurry! Be sure to include the essentials:

- **Light dressing gown** – it will be warm in the hospital so don't pack your fleecy number

- **Backless slippers** – to easily slip on and off

- **Nightdress or oversized T-shirt** – one to wear during labour and another to change into afterwards. A buttoned shirt or nursing top will help when getting to grips with breastfeeding, if this is your choice.

- **Lip balm** – your lips will quickly dry out during labour

- **Drinks and snacks** – for you during labour and your partner generally (if you're in hospital they will feed you, but not your partner). Cereal/energy bars and isotonic drinks are good to keep energy levels up.

- **Books/tablet/magazines/phone** – to keep you entertained

- **A change of clothes** – to wear home

- **Clothes for baby** – two to three sleepsuits or vests, socks or booties, scratch mittens, a hat, blanket and a warmer layer if it's winter

- **Nappies** – bring a whole pack

- **Muslin squares** – to mop up any vomit

- **You will also need** – your birth plan and maternity notes, breast pads, maternity pads, several pairs of underwear, nursing bra, toiletries and a towel, water in a spray bottle or a handheld fan may be useful if it's warm and, if you're in hospital, an eye mask and earplugs may be useful for a potentially noisy maternity ward.

YOUR NOTES

....
....
....
....
....
....
....
....
....
....
....
....
....
....

YOUR NOTES

....

....

....

....

....

....

....

....

....

....

....

....

....

....

....

....

THE FIRST
FEW WEEKS

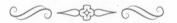

Take these tips on board for the
early days at home while you
are navigating the first stages
of new parenthood. Don't be
afraid to ask for help or say
no to overeager visitors!

DEALING WITH VISITORS

It might be an idea to make some rules beforehand – remember, you don't have to be polite and let everyone through your front door as soon as you get home from the hospital. Many friends and family members will be keen to see you and the new arrival, but it's OK to put them off. You may not want any visitors at all in the first few days (perhaps even weeks!) while you find your feet, and the last thing you want is to be making endless cups of tea for other people. Or perhaps you'll want to make an exception for family and allow your nearest and dearest to visit during those early days. Find the confidence to tell people they are welcome to visit, but should keep it short, perhaps staying only for an hour. In some cultures, visitors are frowned upon for the first two weeks of a baby's life while new parents get to grips with things. Have a chat with your partner, come to an agreement about how to deal with the potential influx of visitors and stick with it if you can.

ACCEPTING HELP

When the visitors do start to descend, it's likely that some of them will offer help or ask if they can bring you anything. Don't feel you have to refuse out of politeness – they're offering because they want to help make your life easier. If they offer to make the tea, let them – not everyone will. If they ask if they can pick anything up for you on the way over, don't be afraid to give them a short shopping list

– they offered, after all! Or if they want to bring you a prepared meal – accept enthusiastically. If some wonderful visitor wants to run a duster or hoover around your home for you – say yes please! And if some saintly being offers to watch the baby for an hour while you have a quick nap – bite their hand off! These offers will be, at best, few and far between, so don't turn them down lightly.

GETTING OUT
OF THE HOUSE

The thought of leaving the house with your baby in the first few weeks might seem rather daunting – suddenly you need to think about carrying around rather a lot of kit so that you are prepared for every eventuality. In reality all you really need at this stage is changing equipment, something to feed the baby if you are bottle-feeding and a change of baby clothes. You will soon work out what you need to have with you each time you leave the house – this parenting lark is an endless learning curve after all. If you find yourself spending the whole day at home, try to get outside if only for a breath of fresh air and a walk around the block. The fresh air is good for the baby too and the motion of the buggy can help get them to sleep. If you find yourself staying at home for days on end you might begin to feel quite isolated so getting outside is important. Give yourself something to do, whether that involves heading to the shop for milk and bread or grabbing a takeaway coffee (you could probably use the caffeine!) and walking around the park with it. Get your partner out too – it will do you both the world of good and the exercise will boost your mood and make your rather tired self feel a lot more alert.

CATCHING SLEEP WHERE YOU CAN

In the weeks leading up to the arrival it can be a good idea to practise sleeping for short periods of time. The art of power napping should not be undervalued and, once the baby arrives, you'll want to be ready to grab that shut-eye whenever a small window of opportunity presents itself. Before the big day arrives, if you're feeling fatigued and have somewhere between 30 minutes and an hour to spare during the day, take yourself to bed – use an eye mask if you think it will help –

clear your mind and attempt to sleep for a short while. Set an alarm so you achieve the "power" part of your nap – and so that you don't oversleep and potentially ruin your night-time rest. Once your baby arrives, you'll be grateful that you're able to snatch these small pockets of sleep wherever you can – when and if your baby decides to sleep. If there are two of you caring for your baby, and you're both on leave at least for the first few weeks, it's a good idea to take it in turns to watch the baby while the other catches up on sleep, whenever possible.

PRACTICAL TIPS
FOR AN EASIER LIFE

◆ **Online shopping** – don't bother trying to do a big food shop during the first few weeks. Order groceries online and have them brought to your door. The same goes for baby gear that you might be lacking – many retailers offer next-day delivery if, for example, you need those extra muslins quickly, and you might even find some supermarkets will bring them with your food shop.

◆ **Easy meals** – hopefully you had time to batch cook some dinners before your baby arrived, so your freezer should be heaving with tasty meals. However, you will soon blitz your way through these, so it's worth finding some easy, quick and nutritious meals that you can whip up in minutes when the last thing you feel like doing is cooking.

◆ **Washing** – you might find the washing machine is permanently switched on in the early days as your baby wreaks havoc over clothes, muslins, blankets, your clothes, and so on. Think ahead about the time of year and prepare accordingly when it comes to drying all of these things quickly and effectively. Perhaps you can hang washing outside, but, if the season dictates otherwise and you don't want to use the tumble dryer endlessly, invest in a heated drying rack to speed up the process.

YOUR NOTES

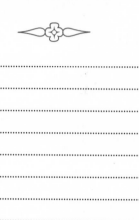

....
....
....
....
....
....
....
....
....
....
....
....
....
....

YOUR NOTES

....
....
....
....
....
....
....
....
....
....
....
....
....
....
....
....

FEEDING
YOUR BABY

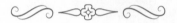

Babies need to feed A LOT, which
can make doing it successfully
a daunting task. Just remember
that, whether you choose to
bottle-feed or breastfeed, there
is help and support out there.

Ah, babies! They're more than just adorable little creatures on whom you can blame your farts.

TINA FEY

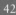

BREASTMILK vs FORMULA

The choice you make about how to feed your baby is a very personal one and it all boils down to what feels right for you. Here is a list of pros and cons to help you make your decision:

Breastmilk

Pros:

◆ It doesn't cost anything

◆ It is designed specifically for your baby

◆ It protects your baby against illnesses.

Cons:

◆ Only the mother can do it (unless you also express)

◆ It might take a while for both Mum and baby to get to grips with

◆ It might take a while to get used to feeding when out and about.

Ask your midwife or health visitor for more information about breastfeeding.

Formula

Pros:

◆ Partner or family members can also feed the baby

◆ It is likely to be more comfortable for the mother

◆ Modern formulas are better developed to meet the nutritional needs of the baby.

Cons:

◆ It can be pricey

◆ It does not contain the same things found in breast milk that are tailored to your baby

◆ Sterilizing bottles can be time consuming.

BREASTFEEDING TIPS

◆ If your baby doesn't feed well in the traditional "cradle hold" position, try reclining with the help of a few pillows or lying on your side with baby on the bed.

◆ If your milk supply needs a bit of a boost, try eating more porridge oats and drinking fennel or fenugreek tea for a helping hand. These are thought to help increase your milk production.

◆ If your baby isn't taking well to breastfeeding, try feeding them when they are sleepy as you may find them a bit more amenable. You could also express your milk and bottle-feed them while you try to rectify the situation.

◆ You may want to feed on demand in the early days to ensure milk production is up and that your baby is getting all the milk they need.

◆ You might find yourself frustrated if you experience breastfeeding issues – but think carefully before giving up – make sure you feel OK about it and won't regret it later. Sometimes perseverance is the key.

◆ Remember it is illegal for anyone to ask a breastfeeding woman to leave a public place. Feeding your baby is one of the most natural acts you can carry out – try to do so with confidence.

◆ Mastitis (inflammation of the breast tissue) can be resolved if the causes are caught early – such as blocked milk ducts or cracked nipples. Keep on top of these issues and also keep a leafy cabbage in the freezer, as placing the leaves into your bra can help to relieve the symptoms. If these symptoms persist, however, you will need to seek medical advice.

BOTTLE-FEEDING TIPS

◆ When it comes to sterilizing your bottles and equipment, remember that everything – bottles, teats, caps, tongs, retaining rings, milk scoops, etc. – must be washed in warm soapy water before being sterilized. Research the different methods of sterilization – there are many options.

◆ Follow the instructions on the packaging to the letter – it is very important that you combine the right amount of formula and boiled water for the optimum feed for your baby.

◆ If you need to make bottles in advance, make sure you cool them quickly under the cold tap and put them straight in the fridge where you should keep them for no longer than 24 hours.

◆ Always fill the kettle with fresh water when preparing formula for your baby.

◆ Don't warm the bottle in the microwave as it heats the milk unevenly – instead place the bottle in a container of warm water or use a specially designed bottle warmer.

Nursing gives you
superhuman powers.

GWEN STEFANI

I see something deeper,
more infinite, more
eternal than the ocean
in the expression of the
eyes of a little baby when
it wakes in the morning
and coos or laughs
because it sees the sun
shining on its cradle.

VINCENT VAN GOGH

CLUSTER FEEDING

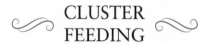

"Cluster feeding" is when your baby has a number of feeds close together – often with only a half-hour gap – and this can happen at any time of the day or night. There are many reasons for cluster feeding, ranging from your baby oversleeping and trying to catch up on feeds, your milk not being as rich at a certain time of day as it is at others, your baby craving the comfort of breastfeeding, or your milk production being a little low when you are tired or at certain times of the day or night. The best way to deal with it is just to feed your baby as often as they want to be fed. If you feed your baby on demand your body will produce the right amount of milk and they will ask you for it! Just look for signs of them sucking on their fist or smacking their lips. Remember that if you give them formula to supplement breastfeeding it is likely to lessen your milk production.

EXPRESSING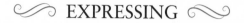

You might decide you want to express milk for various reasons: because your baby hasn't taken to breastfeeding, but you still want them to have your breast milk; or you want your partner to help out with some of the feeds; or perhaps you want to try it to help increase milk production. Or you might decide you want to combine breastfeeding with bottle-feeding and would prefer your baby was bottle-fed breast milk. When it comes to expressing equipment there are several options – you can do this by hand, with a manual pump or with an electric pump. An electric pump will cost you more but is likely to be more effective. There are also single and double models available. If you only plan to express at the beginning to help improve milk flow, consider hiring a hospital-grade electric pump for a month or so before deciding whether you want to purchase an electric model. Do some research into open- and closed-system breast pumps before making your choice.

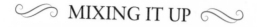

MIXING IT UP

If Mum is finding breastfeeding difficult – perhaps suffering from sore nipples or mastitis (this usually affects one breast, with the breast tissue becoming sore and inflamed), milk production is down, or your baby isn't always as willing to feed as you had hoped they would be – you could try combining breast and bottle-feeding. This is a good alternative to giving up breastfeeding altogether as you will leave your options open, and your baby will still be getting the benefits of the breast milk designed especially for them. Think about what would work best for you, perhaps you want to breastfeed *and* express for bottle-feeding, or maybe you want to combine breastfeeding with formula. Talk this through with your midwife or health visitor to hash out the pros and cons. You might find that formula suits later on in the day or evening, when you are tired or when it is possible that your partner or a family member could bottle-feed the baby, or you may decide that bottle-feeding when you are out and about is a far simpler option.

FEEDING ON THE MOVE

Whether you're expressing or formula-feeding, make sure you have sterilized bottles and either the expressed milk or formula with you. You might want to heat this up beforehand and keep it in an insulated bottle warmer – which should keep the milk warm for several hours depending on its make – or, if you are going to a friend's house, a cafe or a restaurant, you will be able to request some hot water to warm it up when it is needed. If breastfeeding when out and about you might want to consider clothes suitable for nursing so you can access your breasts quickly and easily when your baby needs a feed, and to avoid having to semi-undress or have an awkward tangle of clothes. A nursing bra is a must, and you might even want to consider a muslin or shawl draped over your shoulder and baby or a modesty/ nursing cover if you are nervous about feeding in public in the early days.

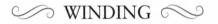 WINDING

Breastfed babies usually swallow less air than bottle-fed babies, but, regardless of how your baby feeds, it can be useful to know how to coax out that trapped air. This can help prevent colic and discomfort as well as the baby bringing up some of their feed. Anti-colic teats are available for bottles to reduce the amount of air your baby takes in when bottle-feeding, and sitting the baby up when feeding can also help as will burping them halfway through a feed. When breastfeeding, burp your baby when you change sides to avoid any air becoming trapped and causing them discomfort. You will learn to spot the signs when your baby needs burping or is suffering from trapped wind that needs releasing. You can wind your baby by holding them with their chin on your shoulder while you rub or pat their back; or by sitting them on your knee facing away from you, with your hand beneath their chin, while you rub or gently pat their back.

YOUR NOTES

....
....
....
....
....
....
....
....
....
....
....
....
....
....
....
....
....

YOUR NOTES

....
....
....
....
....
....
....
....
....
....
....
....
....
....
....

CARING FOR YOUR BABY

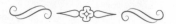

From clothing and bathing, to
nappies and what should be
included in baby's first-aid kit.
Follow these tips and make
the big decisions about the
nappies that work for you.

Children don't think
about yesterday and
they don't think about
tomorrow, they just
exist in the moment.

Jessalyn Gilsig

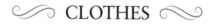

CLOTHES

When it comes to clothes, think about your baby's due date and plan accordingly. This is really just a case of common sense. For example, if your baby is due at the height of summer and you are used to particularly hot temperatures, then it's likely you won't need a snowsuit to fit a newborn! However, a winter baby will definitely need more in the way of layers – so plenty of vests, onesies/Babygros with feet (this is especially important as baby socks get lost easily), and cardigans or jackets. And due to the general amount of mess your bundle of joy is likely to create, you'll find yourself changing their clothes several times a day – so enthusiastically accept those offers of second-hand baby clothes from friends. You'll be grateful for them when changing baby for the fourth time that day after yet another poo or vomit explosion! Most Babygros have folded-over edges at the neck so you can pull these down over the baby's shoulders and body in the event of such an explosion – and avoid taking the mess past their face.

BATHING
⮜ IN THE ⮞
FIRST MONTH

When a baby is brand new, many people prefer to use a simple washing technique known as "topping and tailing", which involves washing your baby's face and bottom with cotton wool from the safety of their changing mat. Make sure the room is at a good temperature. Remove all of your baby's clothes, apart from their vest and nappy, and wrap them in a towel. Take a bowl of warm water and dip a piece of cotton wool into it, making sure that the cotton wool doesn't soak up too much moisture. Gently wipe it under your baby's eyes – use a fresh piece for each eye so as not to transfer any potential infection. Use another piece, dampened, to clean *around* your baby's ears – but *not* inside them – then wash your baby's face, neck and hands using the same method and dry gently with the towel. Remove their nappy and wash baby's bottom and genital area in the same way, drying carefully. Remember with girls you need to wipe from front to back and boys from back to front. For each step, remember to use a fresh piece of dampened cotton wool. There are various options when it comes to baths for older babies – you could opt for a washing-up bowl, a baby bath, or your regular bath if you have one. Don't feel you have to wash your baby every day. There is no need for this and you may find it dries out their skin. However, on the other hand, you may discover that they love it and it helps them to settle, in which case incorporating bathing into their nightly routine can work very well. Don't add any bubble bath or product to the bathwater in your baby's first month.

BATHING
～ AFTER THE ～
FIRST MONTH

When your baby has reached their one-month milestone, you can start adding a cleanser to their bathwater. Always use a product especially for babies – there is a wide range available – but don't add too much. The bathwater shouldn't be too hot – aim for between 37°C and 38°C, or around 100°F – and the water should be about 8–10 cm/3–4 in. deep. You can measure the temperature with a thermometer or get an idea by dipping your elbow in to test the water – it should feel lukewarm. You'll find it easier to wash your baby's face and hair before you place them into the water. Then carefully lower them into the bath (remember babies are slippery when wet so hold them firmly – the best way to do this is to put your arm around their back and get a good grip on their furthest arm). Gently wash the rest of their body, keeping their head clear of the water, and patting them dry with a towel afterwards. If baby doesn't much like bathing, try having a bath together. Climb into the bath yourself and then get someone to hand baby to you. Talk to your baby while you bathe them and it will soothe them, possibly getting them ready for sleep.

The best way to make
children good is to
make them happy.

Oscar Wilde

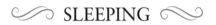 SLEEPING

There are lots of decisions to be made when it comes to caring for your baby and the most important thing to remember is that the decisions need to feel right for you. Newborn babies will sleep for around 16 hours a day and it's likely that there will be no pattern to this at first. Once they reach six to eight weeks they will start to sleep for longer periods at night and take shorter naps in the day. It is often advised that a baby should sleep in a crib in their parents' bedroom for the first six months before moving to a cot either still in the parents' bedroom or in the baby's own room. Some parents like to co-sleep with their baby, which also has its benefits, although it is worth reading up on safe co-sleeping positions and guidelines in order for you all to sleep soundly and safely. For more on sleeping routines and advice, see the dedicated chapter on page 105.

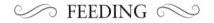

FEEDING

Newborn babies will need feeding as often and for as long as they want. After a few days this will lessen to around every 3 hours – and as a rough guide they should be fed around eight times in a 24-hour period for the first few weeks. There are several options when it comes to feeding – breastfeeding, expressing and bottle-feeding, formula-feeding or a mixture of these. When it comes to this decision the most important thing is that it's right for you. There are pros and cons to all options – breastfeeding is free, on tap and offers nourishment and nutrients designed specifically for your baby, but only the mother can administer the feeds (unless a mixture of expressing and breastfeeding is used); the formulas available these days are packed full of the nutrients your baby needs, but the sheer volume needed can mean that this method quickly becomes expensive. For more details on the various feeding methods, see the dedicated chapter on page 41.

NAPPY CHANGING

Welcome to the world of nappies – you are going to see a lot of them! The average newborn gets through 10–12 nappies a day, while older babies only need changing 6–8 times a day. Some babies have delicate skin and as soon as their nappy is wet it should be changed to prevent their bottom from becoming sore and red, however other babies only need to be changed before or after every feed. When a baby has done a poo, however, they will always need to be changed immediately to avoid nappy rash, which will only upset them (and you).

As soon as your baby is old enough to start squirming you might want to start changing them on a mat on the floor or in the middle of your bed for safety. And always make sure you have the following equipment to hand:

◆ Changing mat

◆ Clean nappy/liner and cover if reusable

◆ Cotton wool or baby wipes

◆ Barrier cream

◆ Clean clothes

◆ Bag for the dirty nappy/wipes

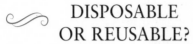

DISPOSABLE OR REUSABLE?

Disposable nappies may seem like the most logical and hassle-free option when you have a million things to think about, but there are other options to consider too. When it comes to reusable nappies, gone are the days when terry towelling nappies were the only option (although these are still the cheapest). These days modern fitted reusable cotton nappies are also available, featuring an outer cover holding a pad and liner in place. These are both environmentally friendly and offer huge savings when compared with disposable. You may decide that you'd like to use both disposable and reusable – in that case, perhaps it would make sense to opt for reusable nappies around the home and disposable nappies when you're out and about. If you're undecided, see if a friend will lend you the outer covers to try out on your baby and you can give reusables a trial run. Don't buy too many nappies until you have met your baby – they come in a variety of sizes and you don't yet know what size your baby is!

AILMENTS TO
WATCH OUT FOR

◆ If your baby has had fewer than three poos in a week they may be constipated. Lie them down on a changing mat and try rotating their legs gently in a cycling motion to get things going.

◆ Baby acne – tiny red or white pimples on a baby's skin – is very common and usually clears itself up without intervention after a few weeks.

◆ If your baby has a pink and watery eye, they may have conjunctivitis – this can be due to a blocked tear duct and can be eased by bathing the eye(s) with cotton wool dipped in breast milk or with a gentle massage to the sides of baby's nose. If your baby is under one month old seek medical advice.

◆ If baby has a cough or a cold, offer them extra feeds to ensure they stay hydrated, and consider using a saline nasal spray, vaporizer or take them into a steamy bathroom to ease congestion.

◆ If you suspect your bottle-fed baby might have colic, try using anti-colic bottles and teats, or consider gripe water if baby is older than one month. Current advice states that you should never give water to a baby under six months old as it will interfere with their absorption of nutrients from breast milk or formula.

◆ Cradle cap – scaly patches of skin that appear on a baby's head – is very common and shouldn't cause your baby any discomfort, but you can try massaging a little almond or coconut oil into the scalp to ease the flakiness.

BABY'S FIRST-AID KIT

It can be useful to prepare for baby's arrival by compiling a small, basic first-aid kit to have on hand should any ailments strike, or should you need its contents at strange times of the day or night.

- **Digital baby thermometer** – to check baby's temperature.

- **Saline nasal spray** – to treat colds and congestion.

- **Liquid pain relief** – usually suitable from two months.

- ◆ **Oral syringe** – to administer liquid pain relief.

- ◆ **Baby nail scissors** – or nail file.

- ◆ **Almond or coconut oil** – to treat flaky cradle cap and patches of dry skin.

- ◆ **Calamine lotion** – for any insect bites, sunburn or minor rashes and skin irritations.

- ◆ **Gripe water** – to sort out colic or tummy issues, suitable from one month.

YOUR NOTES

....
....
....
....
....
....
....
....
....
....
....
....
....
....
....
....
....

YOUR NOTES

....

....

....

....

....

....

....

....

....

....

....

....

....

....

CALMING
YOUR BABY

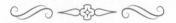

When you feel like you've tried
everything, but your baby just
won't be soothed, try these
calming techniques so you
can get a bit of that shut-eye
you so desperately crave.

Patience is bitter,
but its fruit is sweet.

JEAN-JACQUES ROUSSEAU

DETERMINING WHY YOUR BABY IS CRYING

Before trying out any number of calming techniques, first it helps to discover the root of the problem. *Why* is your baby crying? It's worth running through this checklist to see if any of these reasons might apply. And, with time, you will come to recognize when each of these applies to your baby and fix the situation accordingly.

◆ They are tired

◆ They are hungry

- ◆ They need a nappy change

- ◆ They have trapped wind

- ◆ They are too hot

- ◆ They are too cold

- ◆ They want a cuddle

- ◆ They don't feel well

- ◆ They have colic

- ◆ They are overstimulated

- ◆ They just feel like crying.

The next few pages detail some ways that may be helpful when needing to calm your baby.

SOOTHING SOUNDS

When in the womb, the baby could hear the sound of their mother's heartbeat and so will enjoy being held close and able to hear a parent's heartbeat once more. There are various other noises that go some way to mimicking the sounds your baby will have heard in the womb. For example, you can try a white noise machine, or a toy or downloaded app that offer these sound effects. You may also find that your baby is soothed by repetitive noises you can create around the house – perhaps the washing machine, dishwasher, vacuum cleaner or hairdryer, for example. Many parents swear by music when it comes to sending their baby off to the land of nod, often finding that it will be a particular song or piece of music that works a treat when settling their baby. A good tip is to play the same song every now and again when the baby is in utero, just as you yourself are settling down to sleep; once the baby has been born, when they hear this song, they will associate it with rest time and, hopefully, settle down and sleep.

SOOTHING TECHNIQUES

◆ **Drive in the car** – the soft, rocking motion of a moving car, along with the purring sound of the engine, can soothe your baby, probably reminding them of their time in utero. Many parents admit to resorting to driving their babies in the car in order to get them to sleep when nothing else will work.

◆ **Push in the pram** – if your baby simply won't settle, you may find wrapping them up and bundling them into the pram for a few circuits of the park may send them off merrily to the land of nod.

◆ **Rock in a sling** – bringing your baby close and wearing them in a sling will bring them comfort and may help them to settle. Rock gently from side to side, maybe hum or sing softly, and your baby will be asleep in no time. You may even find you can get on with other things around the house while your baby is asleep on your chest.

◆ **Swaddling** – in the early months, being wrapped in a swaddling muslin or blanket (as described on page 122) can really help to soothe an unsettled baby and get them off to sleep.

While we try to teach
our children about life,
our children teach us
what life is all about.

ANGELA SCHWINDT

REMOVE STIMULATION

A lot of attention and fussing can be too much for some babies and they can get rather fretful if overstimulated. In this case, soothing your baby can be easily done by taking them to a place of calm and quiet, preferably in a darkened room. Blackout blinds are ideal for this purpose. Placing your baby in a crib in a darkened room, with your hand on their tummy as that can help to reassure them you are still there, can soothe them into a calmer (and, hopefully, sleepier) state. Remember that babies are used to the dark and the relatively quiet confines of the womb, so the bright lights and noisy chaos of the outside world can, on occasion, prove a little too much for them.

Children learn to smile
from their parents.

Shinichi Suzuki

CHANGE
OF SCENE

Sometimes a change of scenery can be all your baby needs. Try enlisting a family member or a good friend to look after your baby for a couple of hours – this will not only give you a well-earned break, but might be just what your baby needs to snap out of their crying cycle. Experts believe a new location can be just the thing to help a baby refocus, or become distracted from what upset them in the first place, and change their mood for the better. If there is no one available or willing to look after your baby for a couple of hours, try moving into a different room in your home and spending some time there, or leaving your house and heading elsewhere to change your environment for a while.

Mighty oaks from
little acorns grow.

PROVERB

Parenthood remains
the greatest single
preserve of the amateur.

Alvin Toffler

YOUR NOTES

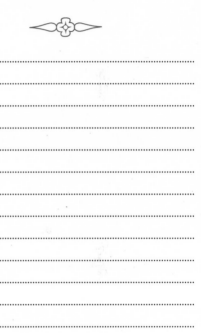

....
....
....
....
....
....
....
....
....
....
....
....
....
....
....

YOUR NOTES

....
....
....
....
....
....
....
....
....
....
....
....
....
....

SLEEP

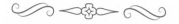

Babies need a lot of sleep,
however at first they don't know
whether it's night or day, and it
will take a little time to establish
a routine. Go with the flow in
the first few weeks and sleep
when baby does – it's important
that *everyone* gets some rest.

A mother's arms are
made of tenderness
and children sleep
soundly in them.

Victor Hugo

IN THE BEGINNING

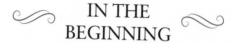

Don't even think about trying to establish a routine in the first few weeks! Newborn babies sleep on average for 16 hours a day – and they will do this when and where they feel like it, with no rhyme or reason other than they need a lot of sleep in the beginning. Being born with little stomachs that need regular feeds means that they will wake up throughout the night, so be prepared to get up several times – but try not to count the wake-ups – thinking about this will only make you feel more tired than you already are! Once babies are six to eight weeks old, they will start to fall into a sleeping pattern that recognizes night and day, and they will also start to sleep for longer periods at night, taking fewer naps during the day. Some babies even sleep through the night at eight weeks, but don't bank on that happening – it's likely your nights will be disturbed for a few months yet. You can, however, think about introducing good sleeping habits at this stage.

ROOM TEMPERATURE

It's important to get the temperature right in the room where your baby will be sleeping. It shouldn't be too cold, but then it shouldn't be too warm either. Ideally, the room should be between 16°C and 20°C, or 68°F and 72°F, and your baby will be comfortable in a light sleeping bag in this environment. Judging the temperature in the room can be a bit tricky, so invest in a room thermometer (you can also buy waterproof floating versions that double up as bath thermometers). When it comes to choosing the room baby will eventually sleep in, think about whether it's colder or warmer than the rest of your home (perhaps it has several outside walls or maybe it's next to the boiler), and make sure there isn't a draught coming through the door or windows.

ACHIEVING A
∽ GOOD SLEEP ∾
PATTERN

Recognize your baby's tiredness to avoid them becoming overly upset. You will soon recognize the signs, which include drooping eyelids, yawning, eye rubbing, crying and comfort-seeking. When your baby is two weeks old you can start introducing the differences between night and day. The best way to do this is to teach them a morning routine where you change their clothes, play with them and take them outdoors, so they associate all of these things with daytime. Taking your baby outdoors will help them to stop producing the sleep hormone melatonin during the day and to instead release it at night when they should be sleeping. When night falls, avoid stimulating your baby, so you can set them up for a good sleep. Stimulation can include, for example, using a night light during night feeds, the TV on in the background, a nappy change or talking to your baby while feeding them. You may want to bathe them before bedtime to get into a regular routine (see page 67). Encourage your baby to nap during daytime noise, so they don't develop into a light sleeper – familiar household sounds such as the vacuum cleaner or washing machine may even help them to settle.

SLEEPING POSITIONS

The safest way for your baby to sleep is on their back with their feet touching the bottom of the crib or Moses basket, with firmly tucked blankets no higher than shoulder height. This is called the "feet-to-foot" position. The on-the-back sleeping position has been advised by The Lullaby Trust as the safest in recent years and has dramatically lowered the numbers of sudden infant death syndrome (SIDS); this is how your baby should sleep from day one. When your baby is a little older, they will be able to move around and find a position that suits them. If you find they have rolled on to their tummy, gently turn them over so they are lying on their back once more. This is good practice and will encourage them to stay on their back in future. Do not worry about getting up in the night to check your baby's sleeping position – this will only add to anxiety and mean potentially less sleep for you – but, if you notice it, roll them over.

SLEEPING TIPS
AND EQUIPMENT

◆ Your baby should **sleep in your room**
for at least the first six months.

◆ When it comes to equipment, you will
likely want a **Moses basket**-style crib
that can be easily moved around the
house, as baby will be sleeping a lot
to begin with and you will want them
close by during the day.

◆ Some parents find the Moses basket on a stand will do the trick for night-time sleeping too, while others might want to look at the other cribs available – including **bedside cots** that attach to the side of your bed to make feeding your baby easier.

◆ When it comes to **bedding**, see page 120 for advice on the safest options.

People who say they
sleep like a baby usually
don't have one.

LEO J. BURKE

The family is one of
nature's masterpieces.

George Santayana

CO-SLEEPING

Opinions are somewhat divided when it comes to co-sleeping (the idea that you share a sleeping space with your baby, so they join you in your bed), with those in favour believing it to be a wonderful bonding exercise that can also help to ease the stress of multiple night-time feeds, while critics say there are safer ways for your baby to sleep. What's important is that you choose the route that best suits you. You might even find you end up co-sleeping for a while without having planned to, finding it easier and enjoying it once you've tried it. Here are a few pointers from The Lullaby Trust for safer co-sleeping:

◆ Put your baby to sleep on their back.

◆ Keep your baby away from the pillows.

◆ Ensure the bedding doesn't cover your baby's face or head.

◆ Keep your baby cool by using a sheet/blanket instead of a duvet.

◆ Make sure your baby cannot fall off the bed or get trapped between the mattress and the wall.

◆ Do not co-sleep if you/your partner are unwell or have been drinking, smoking or taking drugs or medication that could reduce how alert you might be.

◆ Do not co-sleep if your baby was born prematurely (before 37 weeks of pregnancy) or weighed under 2.5 kg or 5½ lbs when they were born.

◆ Avoid letting pets or other children in the bed.

◆ Never sleep on a sofa or armchair with your baby as this can increase the risk of SIDS by 50 times.

SWADDLING

It's thought that the feeling of being wrapped up can help to bring comfort to your baby if they are having trouble sleeping or are thrashing their arms and legs around and struggling to settle. Swaddling goes a little way to recreating the feeling of being in the womb, which is why some babies will find it soothing and sleep-inducing. You can choose either to swaddle your baby using a large muslin (if you are concerned that they may overheat), or to use a swaddling or cot blanket. Here is an easy step-by-step guide to swaddling your baby:

◆ Lay your muslin or blanket on the floor in a diamond shape

◆ Fold the top corner down so the top of the diamond is now flat and place your baby on it so their shoulders are in the middle of the flat edge

◆ Take one top corner and tuck it under your baby's bottom

◆ Bring the bottom corner up and tuck it in

◆ Bring the other top corner around your baby and tuck it in at the neck

◆ Baby's legs should not be straight but able to move into a "frog" position.

If in doubt, there are plenty of easy-to-follow videos on YouTube.

SLEEP REQUIREMENTS

All babies are different and you will quickly get to know yours and what makes them tick. Looking ahead, here's a guideline to how many hours you can expect your child to sleep during the night and nap during the day throughout their early years:

◆ **Newborn** – anything from 8 to 16–18 hours over a 24-hour period

◆ **3 to 6 months** – 8 hours or longer at night (with 4 to 5 hours of naps during the day)

- **6 to 12 months** – up to 12 hours (with 4 hours of naps during the day)

- **12 months** – 12–15 hours (with 2.5 hours of naps during the day)

- **2 years** – 11–12 hours (with 1.5 hours of naps in the day)

- **3 to 4 years** – around 12 hours (your child may have dropped daytime naps altogether by this point, but if they are still napping this will be short and for no more than 1 hour a day).

Loving a baby is a circular business, a kind of feedback loop. The more you give the more you get and the more you get the more you feel like giving.

PENELOPE LEACH

YOUR NOTES

....
....
....
....
....
....
....
....
....
....
....
....
....
....
....

YOUR NOTES

....
....
....
....
....
....
....
....
....
....
....
....
....
....
....
....

BUDGET-CONSCIOUS
BABY SHOPPING

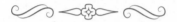

Your baby doesn't need loads
of stuff and what they do need
certainly doesn't have to cost the
earth. Follow these tips on where
to cut financial corners if you
need to and learn how to pare
things back to the essentials.

A baby will make
love stronger, days
shorter, nights longer,
bank account smaller,
home happier, clothes
shabbier, the past
forgotten and the
future worth living for.

ANONYMOUS

BUY
SECOND-HAND

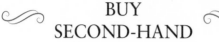

It's fair to say some people go overboard when it comes to buying the latest products and shiny new gadgets for their baby's impending arrival. Don't forget that a lot of what you buy or acquire, you will only need for a matter of weeks. Newborn babies grow very quickly, so any expensive outfits will only be worn a handful of times before they no longer fit. Remember that friends and family members are likely to want to buy the baby gifts – often in the form of new baby-sized clothes, so don't load up on too many new clothes or gadgets for your baby. When it comes to equipment, look for nearly new/second-hand baby sales in your area or try on social media for groups where parents can sell used baby goods. The buggy/pram will be one of the most expensive pieces of kit and it's likely you'll be able to pick up one of these second-hand and in good condition for a fraction of the price. Always make sure to give your purchases a good safety check before use. Some items will need to be new – such as mattresses for cribs, cots and prams, as well as the car seat.

ONLY BUY WHAT YOU NEED

A good piece of advice is to only buy what you need. Do a bit of research ahead of splurging on all the latest baby gear and make sure you stick to the essentials. The shops will still be open once the baby has arrived and, in this age of online shopping, you can have pretty much anything delivered overnight if you really need it that urgently, so it makes sense to buy additional things as and when you need them. You'll save a lot of money this way. See the list of essential items on page 12 to get you started, as well as the list of nice-to-have items if your budget will stretch that far – and if you feel you just can't live without the latest kit.

LOOK FOR ALTERNATIVES

Do you really need that special sleepy-snuggle-feeding-support pillow, hand-stuffed in Scandinavia? Or the newborn snowsuit sporting the latest designer baby label? Or are there cheaper alternatives that will work just as well, if not better, and save you a lot of money in the long run? If there's a particular product you are hankering after, but the price is more than a little steep and paying for it would also mean having to seriously compromise elsewhere, then ask yourself if it is really worth it. If you decide you absolutely *cannot* raise your child without it, then perhaps it's worth suggesting to relatives if they offer to buy your baby a gift. You might find they are able to club together to get you that pillow/snowsuit of your dreams! Or you might see that this wonder product actually has many competitors with the same magic, but at a fraction of the cost, now making it more accessible to all.

SELL USED EQUIPMENT

When buying baby equipment, remember that there is a definite market for second-hand baby gear, so you will find you can sell much of it on and make a small amount back. Some items retain their value more than others – like certain trendy brands of buggies and slings, cots and cribs, for example – so, while you won't recoup all costs from everything you purchased for your bundle of joy, the amount that you do get back will be a nice boost. Perhaps you could put it in a pot/bank account ready for the next bit of kit that your baby will undoubtedly need, or even save it to spend on presents for their birthday or Christmas.

The ideal scenario would be that you have close friends or family members who are perhaps six months to a year ahead of you in terms of child-rearing, and who want to either give or lend you all their baby equipment once they've finished with it. This would save you a good deal of expenditure, so don't be afraid to ask if they are not immediately forthcoming! Some parents don't want to put you in an awkward position – in case you feel you *have* to say yes to their generous offer. They will be worried that you might, in reality, prefer to have some lovely new kit for your baby but don't want to risk causing offence. You could always offer babysitting favours or to buy their gear second-hand if you don't want to just come right out and ask for it. Chances are they will just give it to you or, if some money changes hands, you can be secure in the knowledge that they've looked after the gear and it will all be in good working order.

YOUR NOTES

....
....
....
....
....
....
....
....
....
....
....
....
....
....

YOUR NOTES

....
....
....
....
....
....
....
....
....
....
....
....
....
....

LOOKING AFTER YOURSELVES

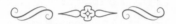

When charged with looking after a brand new person, it can be easy for parents to forget about themselves. Healthy and happy caregivers help to make a healthy, happy baby, so be sure to look after yourselves too!

If your children look
up to you, you've
made a success of
life's biggest job.

Anonymous

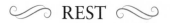

REST

With such a big life change imminent, it's important everyone who will be caring for your baby gets plenty of rest before the big event. Don't plan too many late nights, and make sure you both put your feet up as much as you can. You might both be feeling the urge to nest and get all those niggling jobs around the house done before baby's arrival. That's fine, but plan well in advance to get these things done, giving yourselves a couple of clear weeks before the due date to have some well-earned sofa time to rest and recuperate. Keep your energy levels up with regular healthy smoothies and good, nourishing food, and (try to) take some brisk walks in the daytime.

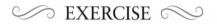

EXERCISE

Both in the weeks leading up to your baby's arrival and once the big day has come, do what you can to boost your mood with some gentle exercise. A simple walk around the block, getting yourself out in that beneficial fresh air, can do wonders and will help you to avoid feeling cooped up at home. As soon as you feel able to take your new baby out of the house, whizz the pram round the block if time is limited, as a minimum, or take a longer stroll to really boost your mood. There are plenty of exercise classes you can join that involve running with a buggy if that's up your street, or mums can usually start postnatal yoga classes at six weeks (a little longer if they have had a C-section), and many classes allow you to take your baby along so you won't have to find someone to look after them.

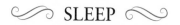 SLEEP

Grab it wherever you can! Before your baby arrives practise some power naps to get you used to having a restful and beneficial snooze in a short window of time. Once your baby is here, you will want to be able to snatch forty winks when they are sleeping or between feeds if a kind friend or relative offers to watch them for an hour or so. With the need to feed every 3 hours in the early days, you want to be well used to reaching the land of nod via bullet train as and when you need to. If you find yourself wired and unable to nap, try cutting down on caffeine (potentially easier said than done), downloading a relaxation/mindfulness podcast and making your bedroom or sleeping space a sanctuary – you might even want to spritz some lavender oil about to help you settle. If sleep is just not happening at naptime, try the relaxation podcast anyway and at least you will be catching up on some beneficial rest.

While we try to teach
our children all about
life, our children teach
us what life is all about.

Anonymous

Babies are such a nice
way to start people.

Don Herold

∾ EAT ∾

To feel good and keep your energy levels up, make sure you are eating well. It's likely you'll be opting for quick and easy meals, but that doesn't have to mean you resort to eating junk and takeaways. Do a little research prior to your baby's arrival and bookmark some easy, nourishing and healthy recipes. Make sure these are things that you like and look forward to, but that won't make you feel sluggish, and make sure they will feature ingredients that are likely to boost your energy levels and help you to feel better in yourself. A good tip is to batch cook some of your favourite meals ahead of your baby's arrival and freeze in portions.

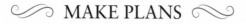

MAKE PLANS

It's important to make arrangements to meet up with people once you've got through the first few weeks and are getting into the swing of things. Above all else, sharing experiences with others who are undergoing similar events can help to boost your confidence and reinforce your coping strategies, as well as help you to remember the value of adult company! Whether you just head out for an hour to meet a friend for a coffee one day or arrange for a family member to visit you at home the next, having things to look forward to and knowing you will have a bit of a change of scene will do you the world of good. Having someone to talk to about what's been going on – and hopefully hold the baby for a bit – will prove invaluable, especially when leaving the house feels like a huge undertaking.

STAY POSITIVE

Being a new parent can be an overwhelming task. Many people live close to their families and have that support network, but others don't. Perhaps you made friends with other parents-to-be on your antenatal course or via a meet-up app. If you are lucky enough to have made some connections, keep in touch and arrange to meet some of them. Even if it's the last thing you feel like doing, you'll be grateful you pushed yourself once you're out and spending time with people having the same sorts of new experiences that you are. If you find yourself struggling with low mood, speak to your health visitor or doctor, seek out one of the many support groups available to new parents, or call a helpline if you'd rather speak to someone anonymously. Try to get out of the house and to be active. Remember, there is plenty of support out there for you.

CONCLUSION:
TEN GOLDEN RULES
FOR NEW PARENTS

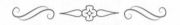

1. **Keep your baby at a safe temperature** – your baby shouldn't be too hot or too cold. A good rule for clothing is to dress them in one more layer than you are wearing.

2. **Support your baby's head** – in the early months when their neck isn't strong enough to support it on their own.

3. **Keep your baby close** – and ensure you have plenty of skin-to-skin contact to help with bonding.

4. **Stay on top of feeding** – to ensure optimum health for both yourself and your baby.

5. **Make sure your baby gets plenty of sleep** – and that you try to get whatever sleep you can whenever you can.

6. **Comfort your baby** – use the soothing tips to keep them calm and feeling safe.

7. **Keep your baby clean and dry** – and follow the tips for safe bathing and changing.

8. **Talk to your baby** – this will help to build a bond with your baby and is a good habit to get into as it will also help with their language development.

9. **Look after yourselves as well as your baby** – it's important both you and your partner get the rest you need in order to cope in the early days. And that you get your rest in order to heal properly after childbirth.

10. **Remember, you're doing a great job!**

If you're interested in finding out more about our books find us on Facebook at **Summersdale Publishers** and follow us on Twitter at **@Summersdale**.

www.summersdale.com

IMAGE CREDITS

Cover images © JungleOutThere (corner scrolls), RJ Design (pram), MG Drachal (bunting), Invisible Studio (text separator)/Shutterstock.com

pp.1, 4, 5, 6, 7, 14, 17, 28, 41, 42, 49, 50, 63, 64, 72, 87, 88, 95, 96, 101, 102, 105, 106, 117, 118, 125, 126, 129, 130, 143, 144, 151, 152, 158, 159, 160 – corner scrolls © JungleOutThere/Shutterstock.com

pp.3, 4, 6, 8, 18, 20, 22, 28, 29, 31, 33, 35, 41, 51, 53, 55, 57, 59, 63, 65, 67, 70, 73, 75, 79, 87, 91, 97, 99, 105, 107, 109, 111, 113, 129, 131, 133, 135, 137, 139, 143, 145, 147, 149, 153, 154, 156, 158 – heading embellishment © Khabarushka/Shutterstock.com

pp.1, 3, 4, 6, 10, 12, 24, 26, 27, 28, 37, 39, 40, 41, 43, 45, 47, 61, 62, 63, 77, 81, 83, 85, 86, 87, 89, 93, 103, 104, 105, 115, 119, 121, 123, 127, 128, 129, 141, 142, 143, 158, 160 – text separator © Invisible Studio/Shutterstock.com